Epigenetics Demystified Understanding the Secrets of Gene Expression

Dominic Jace

Copyright © [2023]

Title: Epigenetics Demystified Understanding the Secrets of Gene Expression

Author's: Dominic Jace

All rights reserved. No part of this publication may be reproduced, stored in a retrieval system, or transmitted in any form or by any means, electronic, mechanical, photocopying, recording, or otherwise, without the prior written permission of the publisher or author, except in the case of brief quotations embodied in critical reviews and certain other non-commercial uses permitted by copyright law.

This book was printed and published by [Publisher's: **Dominic Jace**] in [2023]

ISBN:

TABLE OF CONTENT

Chapter 1: Introduction to Epigenetics   07

What is Epigenetics?

Historical Overview of Epigenetics Research

Importance of Epigenetics in Understanding Gene Expression

Chapter 2: The Basics of Gene Expression   13

DNA Structure and Function

Central Dogma of Molecular Biology

Gene Regulation and Control Mechanisms

Chapter 3: Epigenetic Mechanisms   19

DNA Methylation

Histone Modifications

Non-coding RNAs and Epigenetics

Chromatin Remodeling

Chapter 4: Epigenetic Inheritance   27

Transgenerational Epigenetic Inheritance

Parental Environmental Effects on Offspring

Epigenetic Changes during Development

Chapter 5: Epigenetics in Human Health and Disease   33

Epigenetics and Cancer

Epigenetics and Neurological Disorders

Epigenetics and Cardiovascular Disease

Epigenetics and Aging

Chapter 6: Epigenetics and Environmental Influences   41

Environmental Factors and Epigenetic Modifications

Epigenetics and Nutrition

Epigenetics and Stress

Epigenetics and Chemical Exposures

Chapter 7: Epigenetic Therapies and Future Directions   49

Epigenetic Drug Development

Potential Applications of Epigenetic Therapies

Ethical Considerations in Epigenetic Research

Emerging Trends and Future Directions in Epigenetics

Chapter 8: Epigenetics in Personalized Medicine   58

Epigenetic Biomarkers for Disease Diagnosis

Epigenetic Profiling and Treatment Response Prediction

Epigenetic Therapies for Precision Medicine

Chapter 9: Epigenetics and Society   64

Public Awareness and Understanding of Epigenetics

Epigenetics in Education and Research

Ethical Implications and Policy Considerations

Chapter 10: The Future of Epigenetics 70

Advances in Epigenomic Technologies

Epigenetics and Synthetic Biology

Potential Discoveries and Breakthroughs in Epigenetics

Conclusion: Unraveling the Secrets of Gene Expression through Epigenetics 77

Chapter 1: Introduction to Epigenetics

What is Epigenetics?

Epigenetics is a fascinating field of study that has revolutionized our understanding of gene expression and inheritance. In this subchapter, we will delve into the world of epigenetics, demystifying its concepts and shedding light on its profound implications for genetics and genomics.

At its core, epigenetics refers to the study of heritable changes in gene expression that do not involve alterations to the underlying DNA sequence. It explores how environmental factors and lifestyle choices can influence gene activity and subsequently affect our health and development. Epigenetic modifications act as switches, turning genes on or off, and thus playing a critical role in determining an individual's traits and susceptibility to diseases.

One of the key mechanisms of epigenetic regulation is DNA methylation, a process where methyl groups attach to specific regions of DNA, marking them as "silent" and preventing gene expression. Another mechanism is histone modification, where proteins called histones, around which DNA is wound, undergo chemical changes that either promote or inhibit gene activity. These epigenetic marks can be passed on from one generation to another, leading to the inheritance of certain traits or diseases.

Epigenetics also challenges the long-held belief that our genetic destiny is fixed and unchangeable. It reveals that our genes are not our fate, and that our lifestyle choices can have a profound impact on our gene expression and overall health. Studies have shown that factors such as diet, stress, exercise, and exposure to toxins can all influence epigenetic modifications.

Understanding epigenetics has far-reaching implications for personalized medicine and disease prevention. By unraveling the epigenetic changes associated with various diseases, scientists can develop targeted therapies and interventions to reverse or mitigate these alterations. Furthermore, epigenetic research has shed light on the interplay between nature and nurture, providing valuable insights into how our environment can shape our genetic potential.

In conclusion, epigenetics is a groundbreaking field that has revolutionized our understanding of gene expression and inheritance. It highlights the role of environmental factors in shaping our genes and challenges the idea that our genetic destiny is fixed. By unraveling the mechanisms of epigenetic regulation, scientists are paving the way for personalized medicine and disease prevention. Epigenetics truly holds the key to unlocking the secrets of gene expression and has the potential to transform our understanding of genetics and genomics.

Historical Overview of Epigenetics Research

Epigenetics, the study of heritable changes in gene expression that do not involve alterations to the underlying DNA sequence, has revolutionized our understanding of genetics and genomics. This subchapter aims to provide a brief historical overview of the key milestones in epigenetics research, from its early beginnings to the cutting-edge discoveries of today.

The roots of epigenetics can be traced back to the mid-20th century when scientists first began to question the prevailing belief that genes alone determined an organism's traits. In the 1940s, Conrad Waddington coined the term "epigenetics" to describe the interactions between genes and their environment during development. However, it wasn't until the 1970s that the field gained traction with the discovery of DNA methylation, a chemical modification that plays a crucial role in gene regulation.

The breakthrough came when researchers identified 5-methylcytosine, a modified form of the DNA base cytosine, as a key epigenetic mark. Soon after, they demonstrated that DNA methylation could silence gene expression by preventing the binding of transcription factors and other regulatory proteins. This discovery laid the foundation for understanding how epigenetic modifications influence gene activity.

In the 1990s, researchers made another pivotal discovery – the existence of histone modifications. Histones are proteins that DNA wraps around to form a compact structure called chromatin. It was found that chemical modifications to histones, such as acetylation and methylation, could either activate or repress gene expression by altering the accessibility of the DNA to transcriptional machinery.

The advent of high-throughput sequencing technologies in the 21st century propelled epigenetics research to new heights. Scientists could now map epigenetic marks across the entire genome, leading to the identification of novel modifications and their functional implications. Moreover, studies involving identical twins revealed that epigenetic modifications could be influenced by environmental factors, challenging the long-held notion of genetic determinism.

Today, epigenetics research encompasses a vast array of disciplines, including molecular biology, genetics, and bioinformatics. Scientists are unraveling the intricate mechanisms underlying epigenetic regulation and its impact on development, disease, and even behavior. Furthermore, the field holds great promise for therapeutic interventions, as epigenetic modifications can be reversible.

In conclusion, the historical overview of epigenetics research presented here highlights the remarkable journey from its early inception to the present-day understanding of this field. Epigenetics has revolutionized our understanding of genetics and genomics, showcasing the intricate interplay between genes and the environment. As our knowledge in this field continues to expand, the potential for breakthroughs in medicine and personalized therapies becomes increasingly exciting.

Importance of Epigenetics in Understanding Gene Expression

The Importance of Epigenetics in Understanding Gene Expression

Epigenetics, a fascinating field within genetics and genomics, plays a pivotal role in unlocking the secrets of gene expression. It provides a deeper understanding of how our genes are regulated and how they interact with the environment, shaping our health and development. This subchapter aims to shed light on the significance of epigenetics in comprehending gene expression and its relevance to everyone, regardless of their scientific background.

Gene expression is the process by which information encoded in our genes is translated into functional proteins. Epigenetics, however, goes beyond the DNA sequence itself and investigates the modifications and changes that occur in gene activity without altering the underlying genetic code. These modifications can be influenced by a myriad of factors, such as lifestyle, diet, stress, and exposure to toxins, ultimately determining which genes are turned off or on.

Understanding epigenetics is crucial because it allows us to grasp how our environment and experiences can influence gene expression. By studying epigenetic modifications, scientists have made groundbreaking discoveries regarding the impact of lifestyle choices on our health. It has been found that certain dietary habits, for instance, can alter epigenetic marks, influencing gene expression patterns and potentially contributing to the development of diseases like cancer, diabetes, and cardiovascular disorders.

Moreover, epigenetics helps us comprehend the complex interplay between nature and nurture. It shows that our genetic predispositions are not set in stone and can be influenced by external factors. This means that even if we have a genetic susceptibility to certain diseases, we can potentially mitigate the risk by adopting a healthy lifestyle and minimizing exposure to harmful elements.

Epigenetics also plays a pivotal role in fields such as developmental biology and personalized medicine. It helps us understand how different cells in our body, despite containing the same genetic material, can have distinct functions and characteristics. By studying epigenetic modifications, scientists can unravel the mechanisms behind cell differentiation and specialization, leading to new insights into embryonic development and tissue regeneration.

In the realm of personalized medicine, epigenetics offers great promise. It allows us to identify epigenetic markers that can serve as early indicators of disease risk or response to specific treatments. This knowledge can pave the way for more targeted and tailored therapies, improving patient outcomes and revolutionizing healthcare.

In conclusion, epigenetics is a captivating and vital field of study within genetics and genomics. Its significance lies in its ability to unravel the intricate connections between our genetic makeup, environmental factors, and disease susceptibility. Understanding epigenetics empowers us to take charge of our health, make informed lifestyle choices, and opens doors to revolutionary advancements in medicine. This subchapter will serve as a valuable resource for anyone interested in grasping the importance of epigenetics in understanding gene expression.

Chapter 2: The Basics of Gene Expression

DNA Structure and Function

DNA, or deoxyribonucleic acid, is the fundamental molecule of life. It carries the genetic instructions that determine the characteristics and traits of all living organisms, from the tiniest bacteria to complex human beings. Understanding the structure and function of DNA is crucial in unraveling the mysteries of gene expression and the field of epigenetics.

The structure of DNA is a double helix, resembling a twisted ladder. It consists of two long chains made up of nucleotides, which are the building blocks of DNA. Each nucleotide consists of a sugar molecule (deoxyribose), a phosphate group, and one of four nitrogenous bases: adenine (A), thymine (T), cytosine (C), and guanine (G). These nitrogenous bases form the "rungs" of the DNA ladder, pairing in a complementary manner: A always pairs with T, and C always pairs with G. This pairing is essential for DNA replication and the transmission of genetic information.

The function of DNA is to carry the genetic code that determines the synthesis of proteins, the building blocks of life. The sequence of nucleotides along the DNA molecule forms a unique genetic code that is translated into specific proteins. This process, known as gene expression, is crucial for the development, growth, and functioning of all living organisms.

Within the DNA molecule, genes are specific segments that contain the instructions for making a particular protein. Genes can be turned "on" or "off" in response to various signals and environmental factors, leading to the concept of gene regulation. Epigenetics, a field of study closely related to genetics and genomics, explores how these external factors can modify gene expression without changing the DNA sequence itself.

Understanding the structure and function of DNA has revolutionized the field of genetics and genomics. It has allowed scientists to decode the human genome, identify disease-causing mutations, and develop innovative therapies. Moreover, it has paved the way for the field of epigenetics, which explores how factors such as diet, stress, and environmental exposures can influence gene expression and impact our health and well-being.

In conclusion, DNA's structure and function play a crucial role in the understanding of gene expression and the field of epigenetics. The double helix structure and complementary base pairing enable DNA replication and transmission of genetic information. Genes within the DNA molecule contain the instructions for protein synthesis, and the study of gene regulation has led to the emergence of epigenetics. This knowledge has revolutionized the fields of genetics and genomics, providing insights into human health and disease, and opening up new possibilities for personalized medicine and therapies.

Central Dogma of Molecular Biology

The Central Dogma of Molecular Biology is a fundamental concept that serves as the cornerstone of our understanding of genetics and genomics. It outlines the flow of genetic information within a cell and provides insights into the mechanisms behind gene expression. This subchapter aims to demystify the Central Dogma, shedding light on its significance and implications for our understanding of life.

At its core, the Central Dogma describes the flow of genetic information from DNA to RNA to protein. It states that DNA is transcribed into RNA, which is then translated into proteins. This process is tightly regulated and plays a crucial role in determining the characteristics and functions of an organism.

DNA, the genetic material found in every living cell, carries the instructions necessary for an organism's development and functioning. The first step in the Central Dogma is the transcription of DNA into RNA. This process involves the synthesis of a complementary RNA molecule, which serves as a messenger between the DNA and the protein synthesis machinery.

Once transcribed, RNA molecules undergo various modifications, such as splicing and editing, which further regulate gene expression. These modifications can alter the final protein product and contribute to the diversity of proteins produced by an organism.

The final step in the Central Dogma is translation, where RNA is used as a template to synthesize proteins. This process occurs in ribosomes, cellular structures responsible for protein synthesis. The sequence of nucleotides in the RNA molecule determines the order of amino acids in the protein chain, ultimately determining its structure and function.

Understanding the Central Dogma is essential for unraveling the complexities of gene expression and its role in diseases and biological processes. It provides a framework for studying genetic disorders, developmental biology, and evolutionary processes.

Moreover, recent discoveries in the field of epigenetics have expanded our understanding of the Central Dogma. Epigenetic modifications, such as DNA methylation and histone modifications, can influence gene expression without altering the underlying DNA sequence. These modifications can be heritable and can affect gene activity across generations.

In conclusion, the Central Dogma of Molecular Biology is a fundamental concept that outlines the flow of genetic information in cells. It provides a framework for understanding gene expression and its implications for genetics and genomics. By comprehending this concept, we can deepen our understanding of life itself and explore the mysteries of gene regulation and inheritance.

Gene Regulation and Control Mechanisms

In the fascinating world of genetics and genomics, one of the most intriguing aspects is how genes are regulated and controlled within our cells. This subchapter delves into the complex mechanisms that dictate when and where genes are expressed, shedding light on the secrets of gene regulation and its impact on our health and development.

The regulation of genes is a tightly orchestrated process that ensures the right genes are expressed at the right time and in the right cell types. It is a fundamental mechanism that underlies the diversity and complexity of living organisms. Understanding gene regulation is crucial not only for unraveling the mysteries of life but also for developing targeted therapies for genetic diseases.

At the heart of gene regulation lies the concept of gene expression, which refers to the process by which information encoded in our DNA is used to produce functional products such as proteins. Gene expression is controlled by a sophisticated network of regulatory elements, including transcription factors, enhancers, and repressors. These elements interact with specific regions of DNA to either activate or inhibit gene expression, thereby dictating the fate of a cell.

Epigenetics, the study of heritable changes in gene expression that do not involve alterations in the underlying DNA sequence, plays a pivotal role in gene regulation. Epigenetic modifications, such as DNA methylation and histone modifications, can silence or activate genes without altering the genetic code itself. This dynamic interplay between genetics and epigenetics determines which genes are turned on or off, shaping our traits, behaviors, and susceptibility to diseases.

The regulation of genes is not only essential during development but also throughout our lives. It is involved in processes as diverse as embryonic development, tissue regeneration, immune response, and aging. Dysregulation of gene expression can lead to various disorders, including cancer, neurodegenerative diseases, and autoimmune conditions.

By unraveling the intricate mechanisms of gene regulation, scientists have made remarkable discoveries that have revolutionized medicine. They have identified key genes involved in diseases and developed targeted therapies that specifically modulate gene expression. These breakthroughs have opened up new avenues for personalized medicine, where treatments can be tailored to an individual's unique genetic and epigenetic profile.

In conclusion, gene regulation and control mechanisms are the masterminds behind the complexity of life. They dictate which genes are expressed, when, and where, shaping our development, health, and susceptibility to diseases. Understanding these mechanisms provides us with invaluable insights into the secrets of gene expression and paves the way for groundbreaking advancements in genetics and genomics.

Chapter 3: Epigenetic Mechanisms

DNA Methylation

DNA methylation is a fundamental process in the field of genetics and genomics that plays a crucial role in regulating gene expression and maintaining cellular identity. This subchapter aims to provide a comprehensive understanding of DNA methylation, its mechanisms, and its implications in various biological processes.

At its core, DNA methylation involves the addition of a methyl group to the DNA molecule, specifically at the cytosine residue in a cytosine-guanine (CpG) dinucleotide context. This modification is catalyzed by a group of enzymes called DNA methyltransferases (DNMTs). By adding a methyl group to the DNA, these enzymes can effectively silence gene expression by preventing the binding of transcription factors and other regulatory proteins to the DNA sequence. Thus, DNA methylation serves as a crucial epigenetic mechanism that can turn genes "on" or "off" without altering the underlying DNA sequence.

The patterns of DNA methylation are established during early development and are heritable through cell divisions, making them a vital component of cellular memory. However, DNA methylation is also dynamic and can be influenced by various environmental factors, such as diet, stress, and exposure to toxins. These external factors can lead to changes in DNA methylation patterns, potentially impacting gene expression and contributing to the development of diseases.

In addition to its role in regulating gene expression, DNA methylation has been implicated in various biological processes, including genomic imprinting, X-chromosome inactivation, and the suppression of transposable elements. It is also known to play a critical role in embryonic development, cell differentiation, and the maintenance of genome stability.

Understanding the intricate mechanisms of DNA methylation has significant implications for human health and disease. Aberrant DNA methylation patterns have been linked to various diseases, including cancer, neurological disorders, and cardiovascular diseases. Therefore, unraveling the complexities of DNA methylation may pave the way for the development of targeted therapies and diagnostic tools for these conditions.

In conclusion, DNA methylation is a fundamental process in genetics and genomics, serving as a vital mechanism for regulating gene expression and maintaining cellular identity. Its dynamic nature and involvement in various biological processes make it an intriguing field of study with significant implications for human health and disease. By unraveling the secrets of DNA methylation, researchers can gain valuable insights into gene regulation and potentially revolutionize our understanding and treatment of genetic disorders and diseases.

Histone Modifications

Histone modifications play a crucial role in the field of epigenetics, the study of heritable changes in gene expression that do not involve alterations to the underlying DNA sequence. Understanding these modifications is key to unraveling the secrets of gene expression and how it influences various biological processes.

Histones are proteins that act as molecular spools around which DNA is wound, forming a compact structure called chromatin. This structure plays a vital role in regulating gene expression. Histone modifications refer to the addition or removal of specific chemical groups to the histone proteins, which can alter the accessibility of the DNA and influence gene expression.

There are several types of histone modifications, including acetylation, methylation, phosphorylation, and ubiquitination, each with distinct effects on gene regulation. For example, acetylation of histones is generally associated with gene activation, as it neutralizes the positive charge of histones, loosening the DNA and allowing transcription factors to access the gene promoter regions. On the other hand, methylation of histones can either activate or repress gene expression, depending on the specific site and context.

Histone modifications can also act as "epigenetic marks" that are passed down through generations, influencing gene expression patterns in offspring. These marks can be influenced by various factors, including environmental exposures, lifestyle choices, and even stress. Understanding how these modifications are inherited and maintained is crucial in unraveling the complex interplay between genetics and the environment.

Moreover, histone modifications have been linked to the development of various diseases, including cancer, neurological disorders, and cardiovascular diseases. Dysregulation of histone modifications can disrupt normal gene expression patterns, leading to abnormal cell growth, impaired neural development, or altered cardiovascular function. Therefore, studying histone modifications provides valuable insights into disease mechanisms and potential therapeutic targets.

In conclusion, histone modifications are key players in the field of epigenetics, influencing gene expression patterns and ultimately shaping diverse biological processes. Understanding the dynamic nature of histone modifications and their inheritance across generations is essential to unraveling the secrets of gene expression. Moreover, exploring the role of histone modifications in disease development opens new avenues for targeted therapies and personalized medicine. By delving deeper into the world of histone modifications, we can unlock a wealth of knowledge and transform our understanding of genetics and genomics.

Non-coding RNAs and Epigenetics

In recent years, the field of epigenetics has revolutionized our understanding of gene expression and inheritance. Traditionally, it was believed that genes were solely responsible for determining an organism's traits. However, scientists have now discovered that the regulation of gene expression is far more complex, involving not only the DNA sequence itself but also a multitude of epigenetic factors. One such factor is the involvement of non-coding RNAs, which play a crucial role in the epigenetic regulation of gene expression.

Non-coding RNAs (ncRNAs) are a diverse group of RNA molecules that do not code for proteins. Initially, they were considered as "junk" or "noise" in the genome, but recent research has revealed their significant contributions to various biological processes. These molecules can be broadly classified into two categories: small ncRNAs, including microRNAs (miRNAs) and small interfering RNAs (siRNAs), and long non-coding RNAs (lncRNAs).

MicroRNAs are small, single-stranded RNA molecules that regulate gene expression by binding to messenger RNA (mRNA) molecules, preventing their translation into proteins. By targeting specific mRNA molecules, miRNAs can fine-tune gene expression and influence various biological processes, such as development, cell differentiation, and disease progression. Their dysregulation has been linked to numerous diseases, including cancer, cardiovascular disorders, and neurodegenerative conditions.

Similarly, siRNAs also play a vital role in gene regulation by silencing specific genes. They are often involved in defense mechanisms against viruses and other foreign genetic elements. By targeting and degrading complementary mRNA molecules, siRNAs prevent the translation of viral genes, effectively inhibiting viral replication.

Long non-coding RNAs, on the other hand, are larger RNA molecules that do not encode proteins but have regulatory functions. They can act as scaffolds, interacting with DNA, RNA, and proteins to form complexes that influence gene expression. LncRNAs are involved in diverse processes, including X-chromosome inactivation, imprinting, and the regulation of chromatin structure.

The discovery of non-coding RNAs has provided new insights into the intricate mechanisms of gene regulation and inheritance. By understanding their roles in epigenetic processes, researchers are unraveling the complexities of gene expression and its implications for human health and disease.

In conclusion, non-coding RNAs are key players in the field of epigenetics, contributing to the regulation of gene expression and influencing various biological processes. MicroRNAs and siRNAs fine-tune gene expression by targeting specific mRNA molecules, while long non-coding RNAs act as regulators, forming complexes that impact gene expression. The study of non-coding RNAs has opened up new avenues for understanding the secrets of gene expression and their implications in genetics and genomics.

Chromatin Remodeling

In the world of genetics and genomics, one concept that has gained significant attention and importance is chromatin remodeling. The study of chromatin and its remodeling processes has revolutionized our understanding of gene expression and the intricate mechanisms that regulate it. To unravel the secrets of gene expression, we must first delve into the fascinating world of chromatin and its dynamic nature.

Chromatin, often referred to as the packaging material of DNA, plays a crucial role in gene regulation. It is composed of DNA tightly wound around proteins known as histones. This complex structure not only provides stability to the genetic material but also acts as a gatekeeper for gene expression. The compacted nature of chromatin restricts the access of transcriptional machinery, making certain genes inaccessible for activation. However, through a process called chromatin remodeling, these inaccessible regions can be opened up, allowing gene expression to occur.

Chromatin remodeling involves a series of molecular events that alter the structure of chromatin, making it more accessible or repressive to gene expression. This process is mediated by specialized enzymes known as chromatin remodelers, which can modify the architecture of chromatin through various mechanisms. These remodelers can slide, eject, or reposition nucleosomes, the structural units of chromatin, to create more favorable conditions for gene activation or repression.

The implications of chromatin remodeling reach far beyond basic gene regulation. It plays a crucial role in development, differentiation, and disease. For instance, during embryonic development, specific genes need to be turned on or off at precise times and in specific tissues. Chromatin remodeling processes are responsible for orchestrating these intricate gene expression patterns, ensuring the correct development of tissues and organs.

Furthermore, disruptions in chromatin remodeling have been associated with various human diseases, including cancer. Alterations in the activity or function of chromatin remodelers can lead to aberrant gene expression, contributing to the development and progression of tumors. Understanding these processes not only enhances our knowledge of gene regulation but also provides potential targets for therapeutic interventions.

In conclusion, chromatin remodeling is a captivating phenomenon that unravels the secrets of gene expression. Its role in gene regulation, development, and disease is of utmost importance in the fields of genetics and genomics. By studying the dynamic nature of chromatin and the intricate mechanisms of remodeling, researchers can uncover the underlying principles that govern gene expression, allowing for the development of novel therapies and a deeper understanding of the complexity of life itself.

Chapter 4: Epigenetic Inheritance

Transgenerational Epigenetic Inheritance

Epigenetics is a rapidly evolving field of study that explores the mechanisms through which genes are expressed or silenced without altering the underlying DNA sequence. It has become increasingly clear that these epigenetic modifications can be inherited, leading to the concept of transgenerational epigenetic inheritance. This fascinating phenomenon challenges the traditional notion that only genetic material can be passed from one generation to the next.

Transgenerational epigenetic inheritance refers to the transmission of epigenetic modifications from parents to offspring, affecting gene expression and potentially influencing the health and traits of future generations. While genetic inheritance is well-established, the idea that environmental factors and experiences can leave a lasting imprint on our genes and be passed down to subsequent generations is a relatively new concept.

Research in this field has uncovered several mechanisms through which transgenerational epigenetic inheritance can occur. One such mechanism is DNA methylation, where methyl groups are added or removed from specific regions of the DNA molecule, effectively turning genes on or off. These methylation patterns can be inherited by offspring, impacting their gene expression patterns and potentially predisposing them to certain diseases or conditions.

Another mechanism involves histone modifications, which are chemical alterations to the proteins that package DNA within the nucleus. These modifications can influence the accessibility of genes and, therefore, their expression. Inherited histone modifications can shape the gene expression patterns of future generations, potentially explaining why certain traits or diseases run in families.

The concept of transgenerational epigenetic inheritance has profound implications for our understanding of genetics and genomics. It highlights the complex interplay between genes and the environment and challenges the idea that our genetic destiny is solely determined by the DNA we inherit from our parents. Epigenetic modifications provide a mechanism through which our environment and experiences can shape our gene expression patterns and potentially influence the health and traits of future generations.

Understanding transgenerational epigenetic inheritance has important implications for human health and disease. It suggests that factors such as diet, stress, and exposure to toxins can have long-lasting effects on our gene expression patterns, potentially increasing the risk of certain diseases in future generations. By unraveling the mechanisms underlying transgenerational epigenetic inheritance, scientists hope to develop strategies for preventing or reversing these epigenetic changes, ultimately improving human health and well-being.

In conclusion, transgenerational epigenetic inheritance is a fascinating field of study that challenges our conventional understanding of genetics. It reveals the intricate ways in which our genes can be influenced by our environment and experiences, potentially shaping the traits and health of future generations. By delving into the secrets of gene expression, we can unlock new insights into the complex interplay between nature and nurture, opening up exciting possibilities for advancing our understanding of genetics and genomics.

Parental Environmental Effects on Offspring

In the fascinating world of genetics and genomics, scientists have long been intrigued by the idea that the environment in which parents live can have a profound impact on the traits and characteristics of their offspring. This concept, known as parental environmental effects, is a key area of study within the field of epigenetics. In this subchapter, we will explore the intricate relationship between parental environment and the inheritance of traits, shedding light on the secrets of gene expression.

Epigenetics refers to the study of heritable changes in gene expression that occur without alterations to the underlying DNA sequence. It is through epigenetic modifications that the environment can shape gene expression patterns, potentially influencing the traits passed on to future generations. Parental environmental effects encompass a wide range of factors, including diet, stress, exposure to toxins, and even social interactions.

Research has shown that these parental environmental factors can lead to changes in the epigenetic marks on DNA, such as DNA methylation and histone modifications. These epigenetic changes can then alter gene expression patterns, providing a mechanism through which the environment can influence offspring traits.

For example, studies have demonstrated that a mother's diet during pregnancy can have lasting effects on the offspring's metabolism and risk of developing certain diseases later in life. Similarly, exposure to stressors in the parental environment has been linked to changes in stress response systems in offspring, potentially increasing their susceptibility to mental health disorders.

Furthermore, research has shown that these parental environmental effects can persist across multiple generations. This phenomenon, known as transgenerational epigenetic inheritance, suggests that the environmental experiences of grandparents and even great-grandparents can influence the health and traits of subsequent generations.

Understanding parental environmental effects on offspring is of great importance, as it provides insights into the complex interplay between genes and the environment. It emphasizes the need to consider not only an individual's genetic makeup but also the environmental factors that shape gene expression and ultimately determine health outcomes.

Epigenetics Demystified: Understanding the Secrets of Gene Expression aims to unravel the intricacies of parental environmental effects and its impact on offspring. By exploring the latest research and scientific findings, this book provides a comprehensive overview of how the environment can shape gene expression, offering a deeper understanding of the interplay between genetics and the environment.

Whether you are a student, a healthcare professional, or simply curious about genetics and genomics, this subchapter will provide valuable insights into the fascinating world of parental environmental effects on offspring. Join us on this enlightening journey as we uncover the secrets of gene expression and its implications for future generations.

Epigenetic Changes during Development

In the ever-evolving field of genetics and genomics, understanding the intricate processes that shape our development is crucial. One such phenomenon that has gained significant attention is epigenetic changes during development. These changes play a pivotal role in determining how our genes are expressed and ultimately impact our health and well-being.

Epigenetics is the study of modifications to our DNA that do not alter the underlying genetic code but can influence gene expression. These modifications act as switches, turning genes on or off at specific times during development. They can be influenced by various factors, such as environmental cues, lifestyle choices, and even our own experiences. Epigenetic changes serve as a mechanism for our cells to adapt and respond to their ever-changing surroundings.

During development, epigenetic changes are particularly dynamic and essential for orchestrating the complex processes that guide the formation of tissues and organs. They regulate gene expression patterns that govern cell differentiation, cell fate determination, and tissue specialization. Epigenetic marks, such as DNA methylation and histone modifications, guide the precise activation or silencing of genes at different stages of development.

These epigenetic changes during development are not only critical for normal development but are also implicated in various diseases and disorders. A disruption in the delicate balance of epigenetic marks can lead to developmental abnormalities, such as birth defects or neurodevelopmental disorders. Additionally, dysregulation of epigenetic mechanisms has been linked to an increased risk of adult-onset diseases, including cancer, cardiovascular diseases, and neurological disorders.

Understanding the intricacies of epigenetic changes during development can provide valuable insights into disease prevention, diagnosis, and treatment. Researchers are actively exploring how environmental factors, such as nutrition and stress, can influence epigenetic marks during critical periods of development. By unraveling these connections, we can potentially develop targeted interventions to prevent or mitigate the impact of adverse epigenetic changes.

In conclusion, epigenetic changes during development play a pivotal role in shaping our genetic expression and ultimately influencing our health outcomes. These modifications act as regulatory switches, guiding the precise activation and silencing of genes necessary for proper development. Understanding the complex interplay between our genes and the environment is crucial for unraveling the secrets of gene expression and unlocking the potential for personalized medicine in the future.

Chapter 5: Epigenetics in Human Health and Disease

Epigenetics and Cancer

Cancer remains one of the most prevalent and challenging diseases of our time. Despite significant advancements in medical research and treatment options, the complexity and heterogeneity of cancer cells continue to pose a formidable obstacle. However, recent breakthroughs in the field of epigenetics have shed new light on the underlying mechanisms of cancer development and progression.

Epigenetics refers to the study of changes in gene expression that occur without altering the DNA sequence itself. It involves modifications to the DNA molecule or the proteins associated with it, known as histones, which can influence how genes are turned on or off. These modifications can be heritable and can play a crucial role in determining cell fate, development, and disease susceptibility.

In the context of cancer, epigenetic alterations have been found to be widespread and can contribute to the initiation, promotion, and metastasis of tumors. One of the key discoveries in this field is the identification of aberrant DNA methylation patterns in cancer cells. DNA methylation is a chemical modification that can silence tumor suppressor genes or activate oncogenes, leading to uncontrolled cell growth and division.

Additionally, histone modifications have also been implicated in cancer development. Alterations in the acetylation, methylation, or phosphorylation of histones can result in changes to chromatin structure and gene expression, thereby promoting tumor formation. Moreover, non-coding RNAs, such as microRNAs, have emerged as important players in the epigenetic regulation of cancer. These small

RNA molecules can bind to specific messenger RNAs and prevent their translation into proteins, effectively silencing gene expression.

Understanding the role of epigenetics in cancer has significant implications for diagnosis, prognosis, and treatment. Epigenetic modifications are reversible, making them attractive targets for therapeutic intervention. Researchers are exploring the possibility of developing drugs that can restore normal gene expression patterns or selectively target cancer cells based on their epigenetic profiles. Furthermore, epigenetic biomarkers could potentially be used for early detection and monitoring of cancer, improving patient outcomes.

In conclusion, the field of epigenetics has provided a deeper understanding of the molecular mechanisms underlying cancer. The discovery of epigenetic alterations in tumors has opened up new avenues for research and therapeutic development. By unraveling the secrets of gene expression, we hope to unlock the mysteries of cancer and pave the way for more effective treatments in the future.

Epigenetics and Neurological Disorders

In recent years, the field of epigenetics has emerged as a groundbreaking area of research that has revolutionized our understanding of gene expression and its role in human health and disease. Neurological disorders, such as Alzheimer's disease, Parkinson's disease, autism spectrum disorders, and schizophrenia, are complex conditions with a multifactorial etiology. Epigenetics has emerged as a key player in unraveling the intricate relationship between genetics and the development of these disorders.

Epigenetics refers to the modifications that occur on the DNA molecule and its associated proteins, which can influence gene expression and cellular function without altering the underlying DNA sequence. These modifications are influenced by a variety of environmental factors, such as diet, stress, and exposure to toxins.

Studies have shown that epigenetic changes can have a profound impact on the development and progression of neurological disorders. For example, in Alzheimer's disease, epigenetic modifications have been found to affect the expression of genes involved in memory and cognition. Similarly, in Parkinson's disease, alterations in DNA methylation, a common epigenetic modification, have been linked to the degeneration of dopaminergic neurons.

Furthermore, epigenetic mechanisms have been implicated in the development of autism spectrum disorders. It has been hypothesized that changes in DNA methylation patterns during critical periods of brain development may disrupt normal neuronal connectivity and contribute to the behavioral and cognitive symptoms observed in individuals with autism.

Understanding the role of epigenetics in neurological disorders has important implications for diagnosis, treatment, and prevention. Epigenetic markers could potentially serve as biomarkers for early detection of these disorders, allowing for timely intervention and improved outcomes. Moreover, targeting specific epigenetic modifications may offer new therapeutic strategies for these conditions.

However, it is important to note that epigenetic modifications are complex and dynamic, and their precise role in neurological disorders is still being elucidated. The interplay between genetics, epigenetics, and environmental factors is intricate and requires further investigation.

In conclusion, epigenetics provides a fascinating window into the complex interplay between genetics and environmental factors in the development of neurological disorders. By unraveling the secrets of gene expression, epigenetics offers new insights and potential therapeutic avenues for these conditions. As our understanding of epigenetic mechanisms continues to grow, we are poised to make significant strides in the prevention, diagnosis, and treatment of neurological disorders.

Epigenetics and Cardiovascular Disease

Cardiovascular disease, including heart disease and stroke, remains the leading cause of death worldwide. While traditional risk factors such as high blood pressure, smoking, and obesity play a significant role in the development of these conditions, emerging research suggests that epigenetic factors also contribute to their occurrence. Understanding the intricate relationship between epigenetics and cardiovascular disease is crucial for developing effective prevention and treatment strategies.

Epigenetics refers to the modifications that occur on top of our DNA, influencing gene expression and ultimately shaping our health outcomes. These modifications can be influenced by various environmental factors, including diet, stress, and exposure to toxins. Epigenetic changes can persist throughout our lives, affecting gene expression patterns and thereby impacting our susceptibility to diseases like cardiovascular disease.

Studies have shown that specific epigenetic modifications are associated with cardiovascular risk factors. For instance, DNA methylation, which involves the addition of a methyl group to DNA molecules, has been linked to hypertension and atherosclerosis. Methylation changes in certain genes involved in blood pressure regulation and lipid metabolism can lead to an increased risk of developing these conditions.

Epigenetic modifications have also been implicated in the progression of cardiovascular disease. Research has revealed that changes in histone modifications, which affect the packaging of DNA, can influence the activation or repression of genes involved in inflammation, oxidative stress, and blood clotting. Dysregulation of these processes can contribute to the development of atherosclerosis and other cardiovascular conditions.

Understanding the role of epigenetics in cardiovascular disease opens up new possibilities for personalized medicine. By identifying specific epigenetic markers associated with increased disease risk, healthcare providers can better assess an individual's susceptibility and tailor prevention strategies accordingly. Furthermore, targeting specific epigenetic modifications through interventions like diet, exercise, and medication may help mitigate disease progression.

In conclusion, the emerging field of epigenetics provides valuable insights into the development and progression of cardiovascular disease. By elucidating the epigenetic mechanisms underlying these conditions, researchers and healthcare professionals can develop more targeted and effective strategies for prevention and treatment. Ultimately, harnessing the power of epigenetics may pave the way for a future where personalized medicine becomes the standard of care for cardiovascular health.

Epigenetics and Aging

As we journey through life, the process of aging inevitably takes its toll on our bodies. Wrinkles appear, energy wanes, and our once vibrant cells start to lose their vitality. But have you ever wondered why some individuals seem to age gracefully while others experience accelerated signs of aging? The answer lies in a fascinating field of study known as epigenetics.

Epigenetics, meaning "above genetics," refers to the modifications that occur in gene expression without altering the underlying DNA sequence. This emerging field has revolutionized our understanding of how our genes interact with our environment and influence our health and well-being.

When it comes to aging, epigenetics plays a crucial role. It is now clear that as we grow older, our epigenetic marks undergo changes, ultimately influencing the expression of our genes. These changes can be influenced by various factors, including lifestyle choices, environmental exposures, and even the experiences of our ancestors.

One of the key epigenetic mechanisms associated with aging is DNA methylation. This process involves the addition of a methyl group to specific regions of our DNA, effectively silencing or activating certain genes. As we age, some genes become hypermethylated, leading to their decreased expression, while others become hypomethylated, resulting in increased gene activity. These alterations in DNA methylation patterns can contribute to age-related diseases such as cancer, cardiovascular disorders, and neurodegenerative conditions.

Another crucial aspect of epigenetics and aging is the role of histone modifications. Histones are proteins that help package our DNA into a compact structure called chromatin. Modifications to these histone proteins can either tighten or loosen the packaging, thereby influencing gene expression. As we age, changes in histone modifications can lead to the dysregulation of important cellular processes, which may contribute to the aging phenotype.

Understanding the intricate relationship between epigenetics and aging opens up exciting possibilities for intervention and prevention strategies. By identifying the specific epigenetic changes associated with aging, researchers can develop targeted therapies to reverse or slow down the aging process. Additionally, adopting a healthy lifestyle, including regular exercise, a balanced diet, and stress management, can positively impact our epigenetic marks and promote healthy aging.

In conclusion, epigenetics has unveiled a hidden layer of complexity in the aging process. Through the modulation of gene expression patterns, epigenetic modifications can influence how we age and our susceptibility to age-related diseases. By unraveling the epigenetic secrets of aging, we can pave the way for a healthier and more vibrant future for everyone.

Chapter 6: Epigenetics and Environmental Influences

Environmental Factors and Epigenetic Modifications

In recent years, the field of epigenetics has emerged as a groundbreaking area of study within the realms of genetics and genomics. Epigenetics investigates the factors that influence gene expression and inheritance patterns without altering the underlying DNA sequence. One critical aspect of epigenetics is the understanding of how environmental factors can shape and modify our genes, leading to potential long-lasting effects on our health and well-being.

Environmental factors encompass a wide range of external influences that we encounter throughout our lives. These factors can include our diet, stress levels, exposure to toxins, exercise habits, and even the socioeconomic conditions we experience. Research has shown that these environmental factors can leave lasting marks on our DNA, altering its structure and function through a process known as epigenetic modifications.

Epigenetic modifications involve chemical changes to the DNA molecule or the proteins that package the DNA, called histones. These modifications can either activate or silence specific genes, influencing their expression levels. For instance, certain environmental factors can add or remove small chemical tags, such as methyl groups, to the DNA molecule, which can directly affect gene activity. This, in turn, can impact our susceptibility to various diseases, including cancer, diabetes, and cardiovascular disorders.

Moreover, epigenetic modifications can also be heritable, meaning they can be passed down from one generation to the next. This fascinating aspect of epigenetics highlights how our environment can influence not only our own genes but also those of our offspring. It underscores the importance of considering not only our genetic code but also the environmental factors that shape our epigenome.

Understanding the interplay between environmental factors and epigenetic modifications is crucial for developing personalized medicine approaches and designing interventions to mitigate the effects of harmful environmental exposures. By studying these interactions, scientists and researchers hope to unlock the secrets of gene expression and provide valuable insights into how our genes are influenced by the world around us.

In conclusion, the subchapter "Environmental Factors and Epigenetic Modifications" delves into the fascinating relationship between our environment and the modifications that occur within our genes. It highlights how our exposure to various external influences can shape our genetic expression and potentially impact our health and that of future generations. By understanding these mechanisms, we can gain valuable insights into the complex interplay between nature and nurture, revolutionizing our approach to healthcare and disease prevention.

Epigenetics and Nutrition

In our quest to unravel the mysteries of gene expression, the emerging field of epigenetics has provided groundbreaking insights into the complex interplay between genetics and the environment. One crucial aspect of this interaction is the impact of nutrition on epigenetic modifications, which can have profound effects on our health and well-being.

Epigenetics refers to changes in gene expression that are not caused by alterations in the underlying DNA sequence but rather by modifications to the structure of DNA or the proteins that package it. These modifications can be influenced by a variety of factors, including our diet. The nutrients we consume play a vital role in shaping our epigenome, the collection of all epigenetic modifications in an individual.

Research has shown that certain dietary components can directly influence the addition or removal of chemical tags on DNA, known as DNA methylation, which can either activate or silence genes. For example, folate, a B-vitamin found in leafy greens and legumes, is a key methyl donor that plays a crucial role in DNA methylation. Adequate folate intake is essential for proper gene regulation and has been linked to a reduced risk of various diseases, including certain cancers and cardiovascular disorders.

Similarly, other nutrients such as omega-3 fatty acids, found in fatty fish, and various phytochemicals present in fruits and vegetables, have been shown to impact various epigenetic mechanisms. These include histone modifications, which alter the structure of the proteins around which DNA is wrapped, influencing gene accessibility.

Understanding the intricate relationship between nutrition and epigenetics opens up exciting possibilities for personalized medicine and preventive healthcare. By identifying specific dietary patterns or supplements that positively modulate the epigenome, we can potentially mitigate the risk of developing certain diseases and optimize our health outcomes.

However, it is important to note that epigenetic modifications are dynamic and can be influenced by numerous factors. While nutrition plays a significant role, other lifestyle factors such as exercise, stress, and exposure to environmental toxins also contribute to epigenetic changes. Therefore, adopting a holistic approach that considers all these factors is crucial for maintaining a healthy epigenome.

In conclusion, the field of epigenetics has shed light on the intricate relationship between nutrition and gene expression. Our dietary choices have the power to modulate our epigenome and, consequently, influence our health outcomes. By understanding and harnessing the potential of epigenetics, we can pave the way for personalized and preventive approaches to healthcare, where nutrition plays a central role in promoting optimal gene expression and overall well-being for everyone.

Epigenetics and Stress

Stress is an inevitable part of life that affects us all, to varying degrees. Whether it's the pressure of a looming deadline, a challenging relationship, or even the constant bombardment of information in our modern world, stress can have a profound impact on our well-being. But did you know that stress can also leave a lasting mark on our genes? This is where the fascinating field of epigenetics comes into play.

Epigenetics is the study of changes in gene expression that occur without altering the DNA sequence itself. It explores how our environment and experiences can influence the way our genes are turned on or off, ultimately shaping who we are. One of the most intriguing areas of research within epigenetics is the connection between stress and gene expression.

When we experience stress, our bodies release a hormone called cortisol. This hormone acts as a signal, alerting our cells to the presence of stress. In response to cortisol, our genes can undergo epigenetic modifications, which can either enhance or suppress their activity. These modifications can be short-lived, but in some cases, they can persist over time, leading to long-term changes in gene expression.

For example, studies have shown that chronic stress can lead to epigenetic modifications in genes related to the regulation of the stress response itself. This means that individuals who have experienced high levels of stress throughout their lives may be more susceptible to stress-related disorders, such as anxiety and depression. Additionally, these epigenetic changes can be passed down from one generation to the next, potentially affecting the mental health of future offspring.

Understanding the link between epigenetics and stress is not only important for our own well-being but also for the broader field of genetics and genomics. It provides valuable insights into how our environment can shape our genetic destiny and highlights the intricate interplay between nature and nurture.

By studying epigenetics, researchers are uncovering new avenues for the treatment and prevention of stress-related disorders. By targeting specific epigenetic modifications, it may be possible to reverse or mitigate the effects of chronic stress on our genes, ultimately improving our mental and physical health.

In conclusion, the field of epigenetics has shed light on the profound impact of stress on our genes. Understanding the complex relationship between stress and gene expression is crucial for both individuals seeking to improve their well-being and researchers in the field of genetics and genomics. By unraveling the secrets of epigenetics, we can unlock new strategies for managing stress and ultimately lead healthier, happier lives.

Epigenetics and Chemical Exposures

In the world of genetics and genomics, the study of epigenetics has emerged as a fascinating field that unravels the intricate mechanisms behind gene expression. Epigenetics Demystified: Understanding the Secrets of Gene Expression is a book that aims to demystify this complex topic and make it accessible to everyone. In this subchapter, we delve into the intriguing connection between epigenetics and chemical exposures.

Chemical exposures are an inevitable part of our daily lives. We encounter various chemicals in our environment, such as pollutants, pesticides, and even certain components of our food and personal care products. While many of these chemicals are harmless, some can have profound effects on our health and gene expression.

Epigenetics explores how these chemical exposures can modify the activity of our genes without changing the underlying DNA sequence. It is now widely recognized that certain chemicals can alter the epigenetic marks on our DNA, leading to changes in gene expression patterns. These alterations can have far-reaching consequences for our health and well-being.

Researchers have identified a range of chemicals that can influence epigenetic modifications. For instance, studies have shown that exposure to certain pesticides can disrupt DNA methylation, a key epigenetic mechanism that regulates gene expression. Similarly, air pollutants have been linked to changes in histone modifications, which play a crucial role in gene regulation.

The implications of these findings are significant. Epigenetic changes induced by chemical exposures can affect various aspects of human health, including the risk of developing diseases like cancer, neurological disorders, and reproductive problems. Furthermore, these alterations can be passed down through generations, potentially affecting the health of future offspring.

Understanding the relationship between epigenetics and chemical exposures is not only crucial for researchers but also for individuals seeking to protect their health. By being aware of potential chemical exposures and their epigenetic effects, we can make informed choices about the products we use, the environments we inhabit, and the lifestyle choices we make.

Epigenetics Demystified: Understanding the Secrets of Gene Expression provides a comprehensive overview of this intriguing field, including the latest research on chemical exposures and their epigenetic effects. By empowering readers with knowledge about epigenetics, we aim to promote a better understanding of the impact of chemical exposures on our genes and ultimately, our health.

Chapter 7: Epigenetic Therapies and Future Directions

Epigenetic Drug Development

In the quest to unlock the secrets of gene expression, scientists have made remarkable strides in understanding the role of epigenetics in shaping our genetic makeup. Epigenetics, the study of changes in gene expression that do not involve alterations to the underlying DNA sequence, holds immense potential for revolutionizing the field of medicine. One of the most exciting developments in this arena is the emergence of epigenetic drug development.

Epigenetic drugs are a new class of therapeutic agents that target the epigenetic machinery within our cells. By modulating the activity of enzymes and proteins responsible for epigenetic modifications, these drugs have the power to alter gene expression patterns and potentially treat a wide range of diseases. This groundbreaking approach is particularly significant in the fields of genetics and genomics, where the intricate interplay between genes and epigenetic factors is being unraveled.

The development of epigenetic drugs involves a meticulous process that begins with identifying key epigenetic targets implicated in specific diseases. Researchers then design and synthesize small molecules that can selectively inhibit or activate these targets, thereby restoring normal gene expression patterns. This precision medicine approach holds great promise for treating diseases such as cancer, neurological disorders, and autoimmune conditions, where aberrant gene regulation plays a central role.

One of the major advantages of epigenetic drugs is their potential to reverse epigenetic alterations that drive disease progression. Unlike traditional drugs that primarily target the symptoms, epigenetic drugs aim to address the root cause of the disease by correcting the underlying epigenetic abnormalities. This approach could potentially lead to more effective and long-lasting treatments with fewer side effects.

However, the development of epigenetic drugs is not without challenges. The complexity of the epigenetic machinery and the intricate nature of gene regulation make it a daunting task. Additionally, the potential for off-target effects and the need for personalized treatment strategies further complicate the process. Nevertheless, researchers and pharmaceutical companies are actively investing in this field, driven by the immense potential for improving patient outcomes.

In conclusion, epigenetic drug development represents a paradigm shift in our approach to treating diseases. By targeting the underlying epigenetic modifications, these drugs hold the potential to revolutionize the field of medicine and transform patient care. As our understanding of epigenetics continues to deepen, we are inching closer to a future where personalized epigenetic therapies are the norm, offering new hope to individuals across a wide spectrum of diseases.

Potential Applications of Epigenetic Therapies

In recent years, the field of epigenetics has emerged as a revolutionary area of study in the field of genetics and genomics. Epigenetics explores the intricate relationship between genes and the environment, shedding light on how external factors can influence gene expression. This newfound understanding has paved the way for the development of epigenetic therapies, which hold tremendous promise for a wide range of applications in the fields of medicine and biology.

One potential application of epigenetic therapies is in the treatment of cancer. Traditional cancer treatments often involve surgery, radiation, or chemotherapy, which can have severe side effects and may not be effective for all patients. Epigenetic therapies, on the other hand, target the underlying genetic abnormalities that drive cancer growth, offering a more targeted and personalized approach. By modifying the epigenetic marks on cancer cells, it is possible to reprogram them to behave more like healthy cells, slowing down or even halting the progression of the disease.

Epigenetic therapies also show promise in the field of neurodegenerative diseases, such as Alzheimer's and Parkinson's. These conditions are characterized by the accumulation of abnormal proteins in the brain, leading to the death of neurons. By targeting the epigenetic mechanisms that regulate the production of these proteins, it may be possible to slow down or prevent the progression of these devastating diseases.

In addition to cancer and neurodegenerative diseases, epigenetic therapies have the potential to revolutionize the field of regenerative medicine. Stem cells, with their unique ability to differentiate into different cell types, hold great promise for the treatment of various conditions, including spinal cord injuries, heart disease, and diabetes. However, the successful utilization of stem cells is often hindered by the loss of their pluripotency or the risk of tumor formation. Epigenetic therapies can potentially overcome these challenges by modulating the epigenetic landscape of stem cells, ensuring their safe and effective use in regenerative medicine.

Furthermore, epigenetic therapies may also have implications for mental health disorders, such as depression and anxiety. Studies have shown that stress and trauma can lead to changes in the epigenome, affecting gene expression in the brain. By targeting these epigenetic modifications, it may be possible to alleviate the symptoms of these mental health disorders and improve the overall well-being of individuals.

In conclusion, the potential applications of epigenetic therapies are vast and far-reaching. From cancer treatment to regenerative medicine and mental health disorders, the ability to modulate gene expression through epigenetic mechanisms offers new avenues for medical intervention and personalized therapies. As our understanding of epigenetics continues to grow, it is likely that we will witness even more exciting developments in the field, ultimately leading to improved health outcomes for individuals across the globe.

Ethical Considerations in Epigenetic Research

Subchapter: Ethical Considerations in Epigenetic Research

Epigenetics Demystified: Understanding the Secrets of Gene Expression

Introduction:

In the fast-paced world of genetics and genomics, epigenetics has emerged as a revolutionary field of study. Epigenetic research aims to unravel the complexities of gene expression and its regulation, offering profound insights into how our environment, lifestyle, and experiences influence our genetic makeup. However, along with its promises, epigenetic research also raises several ethical considerations that must be carefully addressed. This subchapter explores the ethical landscape surrounding epigenetic research and emphasizes the need for responsible practices.

Responsible Data Collection and Consent:

One of the primary ethical considerations in epigenetic research lies in the collection and use of data. Researchers must ensure that they obtain informed consent from participants, clearly explaining the purpose of the study and potential risks involved. Additionally, it is crucial to protect the privacy and confidentiality of participants' data, as epigenetic information can reveal sensitive aspects of an individual's health or personal history.

Avoiding Stigmatization and Discrimination:

Epigenetic research has the potential to uncover genetic predispositions for various diseases or conditions. However, this knowledge can inadvertently lead to stigmatization and discrimination. It is essential that scientists and healthcare professionals handle this information responsibly, avoiding any labeling or prejudiced treatment based solely on epigenetic markers. Proper education and public awareness campaigns can help combat misconceptions and promote equality.

Equitable Access to Epigenetic Research:

As epigenetic research progresses, it is vital to ensure equitable access to its benefits. This includes making genetic testing and personalized medicine available to all individuals, regardless of socioeconomic status. Addressing healthcare disparities and promoting equal access to resources will help prevent further inequities and promote the ethical foundation of epigenetic research.

Responsible Communication of Findings:

Communicating epigenetic research findings to the public requires great care. Researchers should present their discoveries accurately, avoiding sensationalism or overgeneralization. The media also plays a crucial role in disseminating information, and it is important for journalists to report responsibly, ensuring accurate representation and avoiding undue hype or fearmongering.

Ethics in Epigenetic Manipulation:

Epigenetic modifications can be induced artificially, raising ethical concerns regarding the manipulation of gene expression. Researchers must carefully evaluate the risks and benefits of any intervention that alters epigenetic patterns. Transparent and rigorous ethical review processes are necessary to ensure that such interventions are conducted safely and responsibly.

Conclusion:

Epigenetic research holds immense potential for understanding the secrets of gene expression and revolutionizing healthcare. However, it is imperative to navigate the ethical considerations associated with this field responsibly. Respecting privacy, avoiding discrimination, promoting equitable access, and transparently communicating findings are essential to maintaining the integrity and ethical foundation of epigenetic research. By addressing these considerations, we can unlock the full potential of epigenetics while safeguarding the well-being and rights of individuals and society as a whole.

Emerging Trends and Future Directions in Epigenetics

Epigenetics, the study of heritable changes in gene expression without any alteration in the DNA sequence, has revolutionized our understanding of genetics and genomics. As we delve deeper into the complexities of this field, a multitude of emerging trends and future directions are shaping the way we perceive and interpret epigenetic phenomena. In this subchapter, we will explore the latest advancements and the exciting prospects that lie ahead in the world of epigenetics.

One of the most significant emerging trends is the integration of epigenetics with other branches of biology, such as developmental biology, neuroscience, and cancer research. Researchers are uncovering the role of epigenetic modifications in embryonic development, neurodevelopmental disorders, and various types of cancer. This interdisciplinary approach allows for a comprehensive understanding of how epigenetic mechanisms contribute to the onset and progression of diseases, paving the way for targeted therapies and personalized medicine.

Another promising direction in epigenetics is the exploration of non-coding RNAs (ncRNAs) and their involvement in gene regulation. Previously considered as "junk DNA," ncRNAs have emerged as key players in epigenetic processes. They participate in chromatin remodeling, DNA methylation, and histone modifications, exerting a profound influence on gene expression. Unraveling the complex networks of ncRNAs will undoubtedly shed light on the intricate mechanisms underlying epigenetic regulation.

The advent of high-throughput sequencing technologies has also opened up new avenues in epigenomic research. Epigenome-wide association studies (EWAS) have enabled large-scale profiling of epigenetic modifications, allowing researchers to identify epigenetic signatures associated with various conditions and diseases. This wealth of data holds immense potential for developing diagnostic tools, prognostic markers, and therapeutic interventions.

Furthermore, the field of epigenetics is witnessing a shift towards understanding the transgenerational inheritance of epigenetic information. Recent evidence suggests that environmental exposures and lifestyle choices can induce epigenetic modifications that persist across generations. By unraveling the mechanisms behind transgenerational epigenetic inheritance, we can gain insights into the interplay between genetics and the environment, ultimately leading to strategies for preventing or mitigating the impact of epigenetic changes on future generations.

In conclusion, the field of epigenetics is rapidly evolving, with emerging trends and future directions that hold immense promise for the field of genetics and genomics. From interdisciplinary collaborations to the exploration of ncRNAs and the use of high-throughput sequencing technologies, epigenetics is transforming our understanding of gene expression and disease development. By staying abreast of these advancements, we can unlock the secrets of epigenetics and harness its potential for improving human health and well-being.

Chapter 8: Epigenetics in Personalized Medicine

Epigenetic Biomarkers for Disease Diagnosis

In the rapidly advancing field of genetics and genomics, epigenetics has emerged as a key player in understanding the secrets of gene expression. Epigenetic modifications refer to changes in gene activity that do not involve alterations in the DNA sequence itself but rather modifications to the structure of the DNA or its associated proteins. These modifications can have profound effects on gene expression and have been linked to various diseases, making them invaluable biomarkers for disease diagnosis.

Epigenetic biomarkers provide a unique opportunity to detect diseases at their earliest stages, even before symptoms become apparent. By analyzing specific epigenetic modifications, scientists and healthcare professionals can identify patterns that are characteristic of certain diseases. These biomarkers can be detected through non-invasive methods such as blood or tissue samples, making diagnosis more accessible and convenient for patients.

One of the most promising applications of epigenetic biomarkers is in cancer diagnosis. The abnormal methylation patterns observed in cancer cells can be used to differentiate between cancerous and healthy cells, enabling early detection and personalized treatment strategies. Epigenetic biomarkers have also shown potential in predicting the prognosis of cancer patients, helping healthcare professionals tailor treatment plans to individual needs.

Beyond cancer, epigenetic biomarkers have shown promise in diagnosing a wide range of diseases, including neurodegenerative disorders, cardiovascular diseases, and autoimmune conditions. In neurodegenerative diseases like Alzheimer's and Parkinson's, specific epigenetic modifications have been identified, providing insights into disease mechanisms and offering potential targets for therapeutic interventions.

Moreover, epigenetic biomarkers hold great potential in predicting an individual's response to certain drugs, allowing for personalized medicine approaches. By analyzing an individual's epigenetic profile, healthcare professionals can identify those who are more likely to respond positively to a particular treatment, minimizing adverse side effects and optimizing therapeutic outcomes.

As our understanding of epigenetics continues to evolve, the discovery and validation of new epigenetic biomarkers will revolutionize disease diagnosis and treatment. The integration of epigenetic information with traditional genetic and clinical data will pave the way for precision medicine, where treatments can be tailored to each patient's unique genetic and epigenetic profile.

In conclusion, epigenetic biomarkers offer exciting possibilities for disease diagnosis across various medical fields. Their non-invasive nature and ability to detect diseases at early stages make them invaluable tools in improving patient outcomes. As we delve deeper into the mysteries of gene expression, harnessing the power of epigenetics will undoubtedly transform the way we diagnose and treat diseases in the future.

Epigenetic Profiling and Treatment Response Prediction

In the fascinating world of genetics and genomics, our understanding of gene expression and its regulation has taken a significant leap forward with the emergence of epigenetics. Epigenetics, often referred to as the "second code" of the genome, explores the intricate mechanisms that control gene activity and play a pivotal role in shaping our health and development. One of the most promising applications of epigenetics is in the field of treatment response prediction.

Epigenetic profiling offers a unique perspective on how our genes are influenced by external factors and environmental exposures. By examining the chemical modifications of DNA and the associated proteins that control gene expression, researchers can gain insights into the underlying mechanisms that determine an individual's response to treatment. This profiling allows for a more personalized approach to medicine, ensuring that treatments are tailored to each patient's unique genetic makeup.

One of the key advantages of using epigenetic profiling in treatment response prediction is its ability to detect subtle changes in gene expression that traditional genetic testing may miss. By analyzing the epigenetic marks, such as DNA methylation and histone modifications, researchers can identify specific patterns that are associated with different treatment outcomes. This information can help healthcare providers choose the most effective therapies for their patients, improving treatment response rates and minimizing adverse reactions.

Moreover, epigenetic profiling holds great promise in predicting treatment response in various medical fields, including cancer, mental health disorders, and autoimmune diseases. In cancer, for example, specific DNA methylation patterns have been linked to drug resistance or sensitivity, allowing oncologists to select the most appropriate chemotherapy regimen. Similarly, in mental health disorders, epigenetic marks have been associated with treatment response to antidepressants and antipsychotics, aiding in the development of personalized treatment plans.

While epigenetic profiling is still a relatively new field, its potential impact on treatment response prediction cannot be overstated. As research continues to uncover more about the intricate interplay between our genes and the environment, the door to personalized medicine opens wider. By understanding and harnessing the power of epigenetics, we can move towards a future where treatments are not only more effective but also tailored to each individual's unique genetic profile.

In conclusion, epigenetic profiling has emerged as a powerful tool in the field of genetics and genomics, allowing us to predict treatment response with greater accuracy. By analyzing the chemical modifications that control gene expression, researchers can uncover valuable insights into individual variations in treatment outcomes. The potential applications of epigenetic profiling are vast, spanning various medical fields and offering hope for more personalized and effective treatments. As we delve deeper into the secrets of gene expression, epigenetics continues to demystify the complexities of our genetic code, paving the way for a future of precision medicine.

Epigenetic Therapies for Precision Medicine

In recent years, the field of epigenetics has emerged as a groundbreaking area of research that holds immense promise for the future of medicine. Epigenetics, which refers to the study of changes in gene expression that are not caused by alterations in the underlying DNA sequence, has revolutionized our understanding of how genes work and how they can be influenced by external factors. This newfound knowledge has paved the way for the development of epigenetic therapies, which offer exciting possibilities for precision medicine.

Epigenetic therapies aim to modify gene expression patterns to treat various diseases and conditions. Unlike traditional treatments that focus solely on targeting specific genes or proteins, epigenetic therapies take a more comprehensive approach by addressing the underlying epigenetic modifications that may be driving disease progression. By targeting these modifications, researchers hope to restore normal gene expression patterns, effectively reversing the disease state.

One of the most promising applications of epigenetic therapies lies in the field of cancer treatment. Cancer is a complex disease that arises from a combination of genetic mutations and epigenetic alterations. Epigenetic therapies offer the potential to specifically target and reverse these alterations, leading to more effective and personalized treatment strategies. For example, drugs known as histone deacetylase inhibitors have shown promising results in clinical trials by reversing epigenetic modifications that silence tumor suppressor genes, thereby inhibiting cancer growth.

Epigenetic therapies are not limited to cancer treatment alone. They also hold great potential for a wide range of diseases, including neurological disorders, cardiovascular diseases, and autoimmune conditions. By understanding the unique epigenetic signatures associated with each disease, researchers can develop targeted therapies that specifically address the underlying molecular mechanisms driving the disease progression.

The advent of epigenetic therapies has also opened up new avenues for precision medicine. Precision medicine aims to tailor medical treatments to an individual's unique genetic, epigenetic, and environmental profile. By incorporating epigenetic information into the equation, healthcare providers can deliver more personalized and effective treatments. This approach takes into account the individual's unique epigenetic modifications, which can influence how their genes respond to specific medications or therapies.

In conclusion, epigenetic therapies represent an exciting frontier in medicine. By targeting the epigenetic modifications that drive disease progression, these therapies offer the potential for more effective and personalized treatments. With further research and development, epigenetic therapies have the potential to revolutionize the way we approach and treat diseases, ultimately leading to improved patient outcomes and better overall health for everyone.

Chapter 9: Epigenetics and Society

Public Awareness and Understanding of Epigenetics

In recent years, the field of epigenetics has gained significant attention and recognition within the scientific community. However, the general public is often still unfamiliar with the concept and its profound implications. This subchapter aims to shed light on the topic of epigenetics, demystifying its secrets of gene expression and fostering public awareness and understanding.

Epigenetics refers to the study of heritable changes in gene expression that occur without alterations to the underlying DNA sequence. It explores how external factors, such as diet, lifestyle, and environmental exposures, can influence gene activity and ultimately impact our health and well-being. This emerging field challenges the long-held assumption that our genetic destiny is predetermined by our DNA alone.

Understanding epigenetics is crucial for everyone, as it has the potential to revolutionize our approach to healthcare, disease prevention, and personalized medicine. By elucidating the intricate dance between genes and environment, epigenetics provides a deeper understanding of the factors that contribute to the development of various diseases, including cancer, diabetes, and neurodegenerative disorders.

Moreover, epigenetics offers hope for interventions and treatments that can modify gene expression patterns, potentially reversing or mitigating the effects of certain diseases. This knowledge empowers individuals to take control of their health by making informed choices about their lifestyle, diet, and environmental exposures.

To increase public awareness and understanding of epigenetics, educational initiatives and outreach programs are vital. By disseminating accurate and accessible information through various channels, such as social media, documentaries, and public lectures, we can bridge the gap between the scientific community and the general public.

In addition, fostering collaboration between geneticists, clinicians, policymakers, and educators is essential for ensuring that epigenetics is integrated into medical practice and public health policies. By incorporating epigenetic research findings into healthcare guidelines and educational curricula, we can promote a comprehensive understanding of this influential field.

Overall, public awareness and understanding of epigenetics are crucial for harnessing its potential benefits for individuals, communities, and society as a whole. By demystifying the secrets of gene expression and highlighting the importance of environmental factors in shaping our genetic destiny, this subchapter aims to inspire and equip everyone with the knowledge to take charge of their health and well-being.

Epigenetics in Education and Research

In recent years, the field of epigenetics has emerged as a fascinating and groundbreaking area of study within the realms of genetics and genomics. This subchapter aims to shed light on the role of epigenetics in education and research, offering valuable insights into how it can revolutionize our understanding of gene expression and its implications for the broader scientific community.

Epigenetics, often referred to as the "second code," refers to the study of heritable changes in gene activity that do not involve alterations to the underlying DNA sequence. These changes can be influenced by various external factors, including diet, stress, and environmental exposures, making them a crucial area of investigation in both education and research.

In the context of education, understanding epigenetics can provide educators with a deeper comprehension of how environmental factors can impact students' learning and development. Epigenetic modifications have been found to influence cognitive abilities, memory formation, and behavior. By recognizing the impact of these modifications, educators can tailor teaching methods and strategies to better support students' individual needs and maximize their potential.

Moreover, research in epigenetics has the potential to unlock countless mysteries of human health and disease. By studying epigenetic markers, scientists can gain insights into the mechanisms underlying complex conditions such as cancer, neurological disorders, and autoimmune diseases. This knowledge can pave the way for the development of targeted treatments and preventive measures, revolutionizing the healthcare industry.

Epigenetics also offers a new perspective on inherited traits and intergenerational effects. Research suggests that epigenetic modifications can be passed down from one generation to another, influencing the health and well-being of offspring. This has profound implications for our understanding of how diseases may be inherited and opens up new avenues for preventive interventions.

In conclusion, the study of epigenetics in education and research has the potential to transform our understanding of gene expression and its impact on human health and development. By recognizing the role of epigenetic modifications, educators can better support students' individual needs, while scientists can uncover groundbreaking insights into complex diseases. As we delve deeper into the secrets of gene expression, the field of epigenetics promises to revolutionize both education and research, shaping the future of genetics and genomics.

Ethical Implications and Policy Considerations

In the rapidly advancing field of epigenetics, where scientists are uncovering the secrets of gene expression and its impact on our health and well-being, there are profound ethical implications and policy considerations that need to be addressed. As our understanding of epigenetics deepens, it becomes increasingly important to navigate the ethical complexities and establish policies that protect individuals and promote the responsible use of this knowledge.

One of the primary ethical concerns in epigenetics is the potential for discrimination and stigmatization based on genetic information. As we unravel the epigenetic code, we gain insights into an individual's susceptibility to certain diseases or conditions. This information can be misused to deny individuals employment, insurance coverage, or even basic human rights. To prevent such discrimination, it is crucial to establish robust policies that protect the privacy and confidentiality of genetic and epigenetic data, while ensuring that individuals are not unfairly treated based on their genetic makeup.

Another ethical dilemma arises in the context of prenatal testing and genetic engineering. Epigenetics has the potential to revolutionize our ability to identify and modify genes associated with hereditary diseases. While this offers the possibility of preventing or treating debilitating conditions, it also raises ethical questions about the limits of genetic intervention. We must carefully consider the implications of altering the genetic landscape and the potential unintended consequences that may arise from such interventions. Policies need to be in place to ensure that genetic engineering is used responsibly, with a focus on promoting the well-being of individuals and society as a whole.

Furthermore, the equitable distribution of epigenetic knowledge and resources is a critical policy consideration. Access to genetic testing, epigenetic therapies, and personalized medicine should not be limited to the privileged few. It is imperative to develop policies that promote equal access and affordability, ensuring that the benefits of epigenetic advancements are widely accessible and not limited by socioeconomic or geographic factors.

In addressing these ethical challenges, collaboration between scientists, policymakers, and ethicists is essential. Open dialogue and interdisciplinary cooperation can help formulate guidelines and policies that strike a balance between scientific progress and ethical considerations. By promoting transparency, accountability, and inclusivity, we can harness the potential of epigenetics while safeguarding individual rights and societal well-being.

In conclusion, the field of epigenetics holds immense promise for understanding gene expression and its impact on our lives. However, it is crucial to approach this knowledge with ethical sensitivity and establish policies that protect individuals, promote equality, and ensure responsible use of genetic information. By addressing the ethical implications and policy considerations, we can navigate the complexities of epigenetics and pave the way for a future where genetic advancements benefit all of humanity.

Chapter 10: The Future of Epigenetics

Advances in Epigenomic Technologies

In recent years, the field of epigenetics has witnessed remarkable advancements in epigenomic technologies, revolutionizing our understanding of gene expression and its regulation. These breakthroughs have profound implications for various disciplines, including genetics and genomics. This subchapter delves into the cutting-edge techniques and tools that have significantly contributed to unraveling the secrets of epigenetic modifications and their impact on gene function.

One of the most significant advances in epigenomic technologies is the development of high-throughput sequencing methods. These techniques enable researchers to obtain vast amounts of data on DNA methylation, histone modifications, and chromatin accessibility. By combining these data with genomic information, scientists can now create comprehensive epigenomic maps that provide invaluable insights into the regulation of gene expression.

Another breakthrough technology in the field is single-cell epigenomics. Traditional epigenomic analyses often involve pooling cells together, potentially masking cellular heterogeneity. However, single-cell epigenomic approaches allow researchers to study individual cells, providing a deeper understanding of cellular diversity and its impact on gene expression patterns. This advancement has opened up new avenues for studying development, disease progression, and even personalized medicine.

Furthermore, the emergence of genome editing tools, such as CRISPR-Cas9, has revolutionized the study of epigenetics. Researchers can now precisely modify epigenetic marks on specific genomic regions, enabling them to investigate the causal relationship between epigenetic modifications and gene expression changes. This powerful technology has the potential to unlock the mechanisms underlying various diseases and may pave the way for targeted therapies.

In addition to these technological advancements, bioinformatics tools have also played a crucial role in the analysis and interpretation of epigenomic data. These tools allow researchers to integrate multiple layers of omics data, including genomics, transcriptomics, and epigenomics, to gain a holistic understanding of gene regulation. Moreover, machine learning algorithms have been employed to predict regulatory elements and identify novel epigenetic biomarkers.

The advances in epigenomic technologies have not only expanded our knowledge of gene expression regulation but also hold great promise for clinical applications. Epigenetic modifications have been linked to numerous diseases, including cancer, neurological disorders, and cardiovascular diseases. The ability to accurately profile and manipulate these modifications offers new opportunities for early detection, prognosis, and targeted therapies.

In conclusion, the field of epigenetic research has witnessed remarkable advances in epigenomic technologies, fueling our understanding of gene expression regulation. High-throughput sequencing, single-cell epigenomics, genome editing tools, and bioinformatics have all played pivotal roles in unraveling the secrets of epigenetic modifications. These advancements not only deepen our knowledge of fundamental biological processes but also hold immense potential for clinical applications. As the field continues to evolve, further breakthroughs are expected, leading to novel discoveries and transformative advancements in genetics and genomics.

Epigenetics and Synthetic Biology

In the rapidly evolving field of genetics and genomics, there is a growing recognition of the interconnectedness between epigenetics and synthetic biology. These two fields, which were traditionally studied in isolation, are now converging, revolutionizing our understanding of gene expression and its potential applications.

Epigenetics, the study of heritable changes in gene expression that occur without alterations in the DNA sequence, has long intrigued scientists. It involves modifications to the structure of DNA and its associated proteins, known as histones, that can influence gene activity. Epigenetic modifications act as a regulatory layer, allowing cells to respond to various environmental cues and determine which genes are turned on or off. This dynamic process plays a crucial role in development, aging, and disease.

On the other hand, synthetic biology seeks to design and engineer novel biological systems by combining genetic components from different organisms. It aims to create artificial gene networks and pathways, expanding the possibilities of what organisms can do. By manipulating genetic information, synthetic biology offers exciting prospects for the development of new medicines, renewable energy sources, and environmental solutions.

The synergy between epigenetics and synthetic biology lies in their mutual ability to manipulate gene expression. Epigenetic modifications can be harnessed to precisely control gene activity, providing a powerful tool for synthetic biology. By understanding and manipulating the epigenetic landscape, scientists can fine-tune the behavior of synthetic gene circuits, ensuring precise and predictable outcomes.

Furthermore, synthetic biology techniques can shed new light on epigenetic mechanisms. Synthetic gene networks can be designed to mimic natural epigenetic regulatory systems, allowing researchers to probe the underlying principles governing gene expression. These artificial systems provide valuable insights into how epigenetic modifications influence gene activity, potentially uncovering novel therapeutic targets for diseases with an epigenetic basis.

The integration of epigenetics and synthetic biology holds immense promise for medical and biotechnological advancements. It opens up avenues for personalized medicine, where epigenetic markers can be used to tailor treatments to individual patients. Additionally, synthetic biology approaches can be utilized to engineer cells that can precisely modify epigenetic marks, offering potential therapies for conditions where resetting or correcting the epigenetic state is beneficial.

As the fields of epigenetics and synthetic biology continue to advance, collaboration and interdisciplinary research are vital. By combining the expertise of geneticists, biologists, engineers, and computer scientists, we can unlock the full potential of these fields, pushing the boundaries of our understanding of gene expression and paving the way for groundbreaking discoveries and innovative applications.

In conclusion, the convergence of epigenetics and synthetic biology represents a paradigm shift in our understanding of gene expression. It offers unprecedented opportunities to manipulate and engineer biological systems, with far-reaching implications for medicine, biotechnology, and beyond. Embracing this intersection will undoubtedly shape the future of genetics and genomics, bringing us closer to unraveling the secrets of gene expression and the complexities of life itself.

Potential Discoveries and Breakthroughs in Epigenetics

Epigenetics, the study of heritable changes in gene expression without altering the underlying DNA sequence, has emerged as a fascinating field of research with the potential to revolutionize our understanding of genetics and genomics. With its ability to provide insights into how environmental factors can influence gene expression, epigenetics opens up new avenues for unraveling the complexities of human health and disease. In this subchapter, we will explore some of the potential discoveries and breakthroughs that may arise from ongoing research in epigenetics.

One of the most exciting possibilities that epigenetics presents is the potential for personalized medicine. By understanding how epigenetic modifications influence gene expression patterns in individuals, researchers can develop targeted therapies tailored to an individual's unique genetic makeup. This could lead to more effective treatments for a range of diseases, including cancer, neurological disorders, and autoimmune conditions.

Another area of interest lies in the role of epigenetics in aging and longevity. Recent studies have shown that epigenetic modifications play a crucial role in the aging process, and understanding these mechanisms could potentially lead to interventions that slow down or even reverse aging. This could have profound implications for the field of gerontology and open up new possibilities for extending human lifespan and improving quality of life in old age.

Epigenetics also holds promise in the field of reproductive medicine. Researchers are exploring how epigenetic modifications can influence fertility and pregnancy outcomes. By understanding the epigenetic factors involved in reproductive health, scientists may be able to develop new diagnostic tools and treatments for infertility and pregnancy-related complications.

Furthermore, epigenetics has the potential to shed light on the origins and treatment of complex diseases such as diabetes, obesity, and cardiovascular disorders. By examining the epigenetic modifications associated with these conditions, researchers can gain insights into the underlying molecular mechanisms and develop novel therapeutic strategies.

In conclusion, the field of epigenetics is brimming with potential discoveries and breakthroughs that have the power to transform our understanding of genetics and genomics. From personalized medicine to the science of aging, reproductive health, and complex diseases, the study of epigenetics has the potential to revolutionize healthcare and improve human well-being. As research in this field continues to advance, we can look forward to exciting new findings that will shape the future of medicine and genetics for generations to come.

Conclusion: Unraveling the Secrets of Gene Expression through Epigenetics

In the journey to decode the mysteries of gene expression, the field of epigenetics has emerged as a powerful tool. By shedding light on the intricate mechanisms that regulate gene activity, epigenetics has revolutionized our understanding of genetics and genomics. This subchapter, titled "Conclusion: Unraveling the Secrets of Gene Expression through Epigenetics," serves as a summary and reflection of the groundbreaking discoveries and potential implications of epigenetics for everyone interested in genetics and genomics.

Throughout this book, we have explored how epigenetics influences gene expression, providing a deeper understanding of how our genetic makeup interacts with our environment. We have learned that epigenetic modifications, such as DNA methylation and histone modifications, can alter gene activity without changing the underlying DNA sequence. These modifications act as a molecular "switchboard," orchestrating when and where genes are expressed, ultimately shaping our development, health, and even disease susceptibility.

One of the most exciting aspects of epigenetics is its ability to provide insights into how our lifestyle choices and environmental exposures can influence gene expression. We have discovered that factors like diet, stress, exercise, and even exposure to toxins can leave lasting epigenetic marks on our DNA, potentially impacting not only our own health but also that of future generations. This newfound knowledge emphasizes the importance of a holistic approach to health, considering both genetic and epigenetic factors.

Moreover, the field of epigenetics has opened up new avenues for personalized medicine. By understanding the epigenetic changes associated with specific diseases, researchers can develop targeted therapies to reverse or modify these alterations. Epigenetic biomarkers may also enable the early detection of diseases, allowing for timely intervention and improved patient outcomes.

While the study of epigenetics has made significant strides, there is still much to uncover. Ongoing research aims to elucidate the precise mechanisms underlying epigenetic modifications and their effects on gene expression. Additionally, ethical considerations surrounding epigenetic interventions and the potential for unintended consequences require careful consideration.

In conclusion, the exploration of epigenetics has revolutionized our understanding of gene expression, genetics, and genomics. It has unveiled the intricate interplay between our genetic code and the environment, highlighting the importance of a holistic approach to health. By unraveling the secrets of gene expression through epigenetics, we pave the way for personalized medicine, early disease detection, and a deeper comprehension of our genetic makeup. As we continue to unravel the epigenetic secrets, the possibilities for improving human health and well-being are vast and promising.